TOXIC RELATIONSHIP RECOVERY FOR MEN

Breaking Free from the Chains of Toxicity: A Comprehensive Guide to Empower Men in Rebuilding, Renewing, and Thriving After Toxic Relationship Trauma

FRED K. FORTNER

TABLE OF CONTENT

Conclusion

INTRODUCTION

In the intricate tapestry of human connections, relationships emerge as the defining threads that weave the narrative of our emotional landscape. They are the promised sources of love, understanding, and unwavering support, sculpting the contours of our lives with shared joys and shared sorrows. Yet, this idealized vision often collides with a harsh reality – not all relationships unfold as the harmonious symphony of companionship we envision. Unfortunately, some traverse a darker path and evolve into toxic environments that corrode the very essence of what relationships should embody.

This introduction is a gateway to a profound exploration, acknowledging the inherent complexities of relationships and the potential for them to morph into sources of toxicity. It is an invitation to embark on a transformative quest toward recovery, meticulously crafted to address the unique needs of men navigating the convoluted terrain of toxic relationships.

As we step into this exploration, it is imperative to peel back the layers of societal expectations and cultural constructs that often shroud the acknowledgment of toxic relationships, especially for men. The prevailing narrative surrounding masculinity can inadvertently foster silence, making it challenging for men to articulate their struggles within toxic dynamics. This book seeks to shatter those barriers, providing a safe and empathetic space for men to recognize, understand, and ultimately overcome the challenges presented by toxic relationships.

By setting the stage for this transformative journey, we extend an invitation to readers to reflect upon their own experiences, encouraging them to challenge preconceived notions about relationships and masculinity. This is not merely a narrative; it is an earnest call to introspection, laying the groundwork for the recovery process that unfolds in the subsequent chapters.

The insights and guidance presented herein are not mere generic prescriptions but tailored responses to the nuanced needs of men navigating the multifaceted complexities of toxic relationships. This introduction serves as a beacon of hope, signaling that recovery is not only possible but an inevitable destination for those willing to embark on this transformative journey. As we navigate the intricate labyrinth of toxic relationships, the chapters that follow promise a detailed roadmap to healing, resilience, and the rediscovery of one's authentic self.

Understanding Toxic Relationships

Definition and Characteristics of Toxic Relationships

1.1 Unveiling the Mask: What Defines a Toxic Relationship

In the intricate dance of human connections, the concept of toxicity is an elusive specter that often wears a deceptive mask, concealing its true nature until the damage is done. This chapter is a penetrating exploration into the anatomy of toxic relationships, seeking to unveil the layers that define their essence and unravel the complexities that distinguish them from healthy, nurturing connections.

The Subtle Beginnings: Recognizing the Seeds of Toxicity

At the genesis of many toxic relationships lies a deceptive tranquility. This section delves into the seemingly innocuous beginnings, where subtle signs of toxicity may manifest. Readers are guided through an exploration of how seemingly normal behaviors can metamorphose into toxic patterns, laying the foundation for a deeper understanding of the evolution of toxic dynamics.

Power Struggles and Control Dynamics
Toxic relationships often thrive on power imbalances and control dynamics. This section dissects the intricate web of control that may manifest in various forms – be it emotional manipulation, coercive tactics, or outright dominance. Understanding these power struggles is essential for readers to recognize the early warning signs and safeguard their emotional well-being.

Communication Breakdown: The Silent Poison
Communication is the lifeblood of any relationship, and in toxic dynamics, it often becomes a source of poison. Here, readers explore how communication breakdowns

contribute to toxicity, fostering misunderstandings, resentment, and a pervasive sense of isolation. Strategies for recognizing and navigating these breakdowns are presented to empower men to regain control of their narrative.

The Mask of Normalcy: Social and Cultural Influences

Toxic relationships can adeptly wear a mask of normalcy, concealing their true nature from both those within and outside the relationship. This section shines a light on the societal and cultural influences that may normalize toxic behaviors, fostering an environment where red flags are dismissed or overlooked. Readers are encouraged to challenge societal norms that perpetuate toxicity, empowering them to redefine their relationships on their terms.

Breaking the Cycle: The Ripple Effect of Generational Toxicity

Toxicity often has a generational dimension, with patterns passed down through families. This segment explores the intergenerational ripple effect of toxic behaviors, providing insights into breaking the cycle and fostering healthier relationship dynamics. Strategies for recognizing and dismantling inherited toxicity are presented, empowering men to forge a new legacy for themselves and future generations.

1.2 The Web of Dysfunction: Recognizing Patterns and Behaviors

In the intricate landscape of toxic relationships, patterns and behaviors weave a complex web of dysfunction that entangles the individuals involved. This chapter is a meticulous exploration into the intricate tapestry of toxic dynamics, aiming to unravel the threads that characterize dysfunctional patterns and behaviors. Readers will embark on a journey of recognition, understanding, and empowerment as they navigate the nuanced complexities of toxic relationships.

The Repetitive Dance: Identifying Recurring Patterns
Toxic relationships are often marked by a repetitive dance of destructive patterns. This section delves into the cyclical nature of dysfunction, helping readers identify and understand the recurrent themes that define toxic interactions. By recognizing these patterns, individuals gain a crucial insight into the dynamics that perpetuate toxicity and hinder healthy relationship growth.

Gaslighting and Emotional Manipulation: A Deceptive Dance
Gaslighting, a subtle yet insidious form of emotional manipulation, is a hallmark of toxic relationships. This segment exposes the tactics of gaslighting, offering readers a comprehensive understanding of how manipulation unfolds. Strategies for

recognizing gaslighting behaviors empower individuals to reclaim their sense of reality and assert their emotional boundaries.

The Isolation Trap: Cutting Off Support Systems
Toxic relationships thrive in isolation, cutting off individuals from external support systems. This part explores how toxic dynamics systematically isolate individuals from friends, family, and other sources of support. Readers gain insights into recognizing the signs of isolation and strategies for breaking free from the grip of toxic seclusion.

The Power Imbalance: Dominance and Submission
Toxic relationships often hinge on power imbalances, with one partner exerting dominance and the other succumbing to submission. This section dissects the dynamics of power within toxic relationships, elucidating the ways in which

control is established and maintained. Understanding this power imbalance is vital for individuals seeking to regain agency and foster healthier relationship dynamics.

The Emotional Rollercoaster: Highs and Lows of Toxicity
Toxic relationships are marked by emotional extremes, creating a tumultuous rollercoaster ride for those involved. This segment explores the emotional highs and lows within toxic dynamics, shedding light on how the cycle of intensity can trap individuals. Strategies for breaking free from this emotional rollercoaster empower readers to regain stability and emotional well-being.

1.3 Shattered Souls: The Impact of Toxicity on Men's Mental and Emotional Well-being

Within the intricate tapestry of toxic relationships, the repercussions echo beyond the surface, penetrating the very core of individuals. This chapter delves into the profound and often overlooked impact of toxicity on the mental and emotional well-being of men. By shining a spotlight on the shattered souls that emerge from toxic dynamics, readers are invited to understand the depth of the scars left by these relationships and explore avenues for healing and recovery.

The Erosion of Self-Esteem: Wounds That Run Deep
Toxic relationships have a corrosive effect on self-esteem, chipping away at the very foundation of an individual's self-worth. This section explores how constant criticism, manipulation, and control contribute to a sense of inadequacy. Readers will gain insights into recognizing the signs of self-esteem erosion and strategies for rebuilding a positive self-image.

Emotional Exhaustion: Draining the Reservoir of Resilience
Toxic relationships are notorious for their emotional toll, leaving individuals drained and emotionally exhausted. This segment delves into the mechanisms by which toxicity depletes the reservoir of resilience, leading to feelings of fatigue, burnout, and emotional numbness. Strategies for replenishing emotional reserves and cultivating resilience are presented, offering a roadmap for recovering from emotional exhaustion.

Anxiety and Depression: Navigating the Emotional Abyss
The impact of toxic relationships extends into the realm of mental health, often manifesting as anxiety and depression. This part explores the link between toxic dynamics and these debilitating mental health conditions, providing readers with insights into recognizing the signs and seeking support. Strategies for managing

anxiety and depression in the aftermath of toxic relationships are discussed, fostering a path towards mental well-being.

Trust Betrayed: Rebuilding Foundations After Betrayal

Toxic relationships shatter the trust that forms the bedrock of any healthy connection. This section delves into the profound impact of trust betrayal, examining how it reverberates through an individual's subsequent relationships and perceptions. Readers will gain insights into rebuilding trust, both in themselves and others, as a crucial step towards emotional recovery.

Post-Traumatic Stress: Unraveling the Threads of Trauma

For many men emerging from toxic relationships, the experience leaves lasting traumatic imprints. This segment explores the manifestations of post-traumatic stress and provides insights into navigating the complex landscape of trauma recovery. Strategies for unraveling the threads of trauma, fostering resilience, and reclaiming a sense of safety are presented as essential components of the healing journey.

By examining the shattered souls that emerge from toxic relationships, this chapter seeks to validate the emotional struggles experienced by men and offers a comprehensive understanding of the profound impact on mental and emotional well-being. As readers confront the aftermath of toxicity, they are equipped with the knowledge needed to embark on a transformative journey towards healing, resilience, and the rediscovery of their authentic selves.

Part I: Breaking Free

Chapter 2 Self-Reflection and Awareness

In the intricate journey of liberation from toxic relationships, the first steps often involve a profound process of self-reflection and heightened self-awareness. This chapter is a dedicated exploration into the transformative power of self-reflection, meticulously designed to empower men in their pursuit of breaking free from the clutches of toxic relationships. Within the sanctuary of this chapter, individuals embark on a transformative odyssey, navigating the labyrinth of emotions and complexities that have defined their relational landscapes.

The Crucial Role of Self-Reflection
At the core of breaking free lies the essential practice of self-reflection. This section illuminates the importance of turning

inward to examine one's thoughts, emotions, and behaviors within the context of toxic relationships. Through introspective questioning and thoughtful examination, readers are encouraged to unravel the layers that contribute to the toxicity, fostering a deeper understanding of their own role within the relational dynamic.

Navigating the Emotional Landscape
Toxic relationships often elicit a myriad of emotions, ranging from confusion to guilt, and even self-doubt. This segment guides individuals through the intricate emotional landscape, providing tools and frameworks for deciphering the complex tapestry of feelings. By untangling the emotional threads, readers gain clarity on the impact of toxic dynamics on their emotional well-being, setting the stage for intentional self-discovery.

Assessing Relationship Dynamics
A critical component of self-reflection involves a meticulous assessment of the dynamics within the toxic relationship. This section serves as a compass, offering practical exercises and prompts to guide individuals in dissecting the patterns of communication, power struggles, and overall relationship dynamics. By shining a light on these aspects, individuals gain insights into the root causes of toxicity, fostering a foundation for informed decision-making.

Establishing Personal Boundaries
Boundaries serve as the armor in the journey toward freedom. This segment delves into the art of setting and enforcing personal boundaries, providing a toolkit for individuals to articulate their needs, values, and limits. By establishing clear boundaries, readers create a shield that safeguards against further toxicity and asserts their autonomy within relationships.

The Power of Self-Awareness
At the heart of breaking free is the transformative power of self-awareness. This section illuminates the profound impact that self-awareness can have on the recovery journey. Through mindfulness exercises, introspective practices, and self-compassion, individuals cultivate a heightened awareness of their own needs, desires, and reactions. Armed with this self-awareness, men are empowered to navigate the complexities of toxic relationships with newfound clarity and resilience.

As men engage with the content of this chapter, they are invited to embark on a journey of self-discovery and empowerment. Through the meticulous exploration of self-reflection and awareness, readers lay the groundwork for breaking free from toxic relationships and cultivating the resilience needed for the transformative chapters that follow.

2.1 Assessing Your Relationship Dynamics

Within the pursuit of breaking free from the suffocating grip of toxic relationships, a crucial and foundational step is to undertake a comprehensive assessment of the relationship dynamics at play. This section is a meticulous exploration into the intricacies of assessing one's relationship dynamics, providing men with the tools and insights necessary to navigate the complexities that have shaped their experiences.

Unveiling Patterns of Communication
Communication forms the backbone of any relationship, and within toxic dynamics, it often becomes a distorted dance of confusion and misinterpretation. This subsection guides individuals through an examination of communication patterns within their relationships. Through

reflective exercises and prompts, readers gain a nuanced understanding of how words, tones, and non-verbal cues contribute to the overall dynamic, unraveling the threads that may have led to toxicity.

Power Struggles and Dominance
Toxic relationships often thrive on power imbalances and dominance. This section delves into the dynamics of power within relationships, encouraging individuals to explore whether there is a healthy equilibrium or a skewed power structure. Through introspective questioning, readers assess the extent to which dominance and submission have played a role, shedding light on the underlying causes of toxicity.

Emotional Highs and Lows
The emotional landscape of a relationship can be tumultuous within toxic dynamics, marked by intense highs and debilitating lows. This subsection navigates individuals

through an exploration of the emotional rollercoaster within their relationships. By recognizing and understanding the triggers and patterns that lead to these extremes, individuals gain insight into the cyclical nature of toxicity, paving the way for emotional regulation and stability.

Recognizing Manipulation and Gaslighting
Gaslighting and emotional manipulation are insidious components of toxic relationships that can erode one's sense of reality. This section provides a toolkit for individuals to recognize manipulation tactics and gaslighting behaviors within their relationships. By shining a light on these subtle yet damaging dynamics, readers empower themselves to break free from the distorted reality that often accompanies toxic dynamics.

The Impact on Personal Well-being
Assessing relationship dynamics extends to understanding the impact on personal

well-being. This subsection encourages readers to reflect on how the relationship has affected their mental, emotional, and physical health. By recognizing the toll that toxic dynamics may have taken, individuals gain clarity on the urgency of breaking free and prioritizing their own well-being.

Through careful examination and introspection, individuals lay the groundwork for informed decision-making and cultivate the awareness necessary to embark on a transformative journey towards healing and recovery. This chapter serves as a pivotal step in the broader exploration of breaking free, providing a roadmap for understanding and dismantling toxic relationship dynamics.

2.2 Identifying Personal Boundaries and Values

In the pursuit of breaking free from the confinements of toxic relationships, a crucial and empowering endeavor involves the identification and fortification of personal boundaries and values. This chapter is a meticulous exploration into the nuanced art of recognizing, establishing, and reinforcing boundaries, coupled with a profound examination of personal values. Through this transformative process, men are guided to navigate the complexities of toxic relationships with clarity and resilience.

The Essence of Personal Boundaries
Boundaries serve as the protective perimeter of one's emotional and psychological well-being. This section initiates a profound exploration into the concept of personal boundaries – the invisible lines that define the limits of acceptable behavior within a relationship. Readers are guided through reflective exercises to discern their own boundaries, distinguishing between healthy forms of interaction and those that breach the sanctity of self-respect.

Setting Clear and Communicative Boundaries
The establishment of boundaries is an art that requires both self-awareness and effective communication. This subsection delves into the strategies for articulating and communicating boundaries to ensure they are understood and respected by others. Through practical exercises, individuals learn how to express their needs, assert their limits, and foster a mutual understanding within relationships.

The Intersection of Personal Values
Personal values form the bedrock upon which healthy relationships are built. This section invites individuals to embark on a deep introspective journey to identify their core values – the guiding principles that govern their lives. Through reflection and examination, readers gain insight into what truly matters to them, providing a compass

for navigating relationships in alignment with their authentic selves.

Aligning Values with Relationship Dynamics

Building upon the exploration of personal values, this subsection guides individuals in aligning their values with the dynamics of their relationships. It prompts reflection on whether the relationship aligns with one's core values or if there is a misalignment that contributes to the toxicity. Understanding this intersection allows readers to make informed decisions about the compatibility of their values within the context of the relationship.

The Empowering Role of Boundaries and Values

Boundaries and values, when identified and upheld, become powerful tools for reclaiming agency and autonomy within relationships. This segment explores how the establishment of clear boundaries and alignment with personal values empower individuals to break free from toxic dynamics. By fostering a sense of self-respect and authenticity, readers pave the way for healthier, more fulfilling relationships in the future.

Through the meticulous exploration of personal boundaries and values, individuals lay the foundation for breaking free from the confines of toxic relationships, fortifying themselves with the strength needed for the chapters of healing and renewal that follow.

2.3 The Power of Self-Awareness in Recovery

In the intricate tapestry of breaking free from toxic relationships, the transformative force of self-awareness emerges as a beacon, illuminating the path towards recovery. This chapter is a meticulous exploration into the profound impact of self-awareness – a tool that empowers men to navigate the complexities of toxic relationships with clarity, resilience, and a renewed sense of purpose.

The Essence of Self-Awareness
Self-awareness is the key that unlocks the door to understanding one's own thoughts, emotions, and behaviors. This section initiates a deep exploration into the essence of self-awareness, shedding light on the transformative journey of turning inward. Readers are guided through reflective exercises and mindfulness practices, cultivating a heightened awareness of the intricacies that define their emotional landscape.

Navigating Thoughts and Emotions
Toxic relationships often blur the lines between one's own thoughts and the influence of external dynamics. This subsection delves into the practice of navigating thoughts and emotions with a discerning eye. Through mindfulness techniques and introspective questioning,

individuals gain insights into untangling the web of thoughts and emotions that may have been distorted or suppressed within the toxic relationship.

Cultivating Emotional Intelligence
Emotional intelligence is a cornerstone of self-awareness, providing the capacity to understand, manage, and express one's own emotions effectively. This segment explores the cultivation of emotional intelligence, guiding readers through exercises that enhance their ability to identify, interpret, and respond to emotions both within themselves and others. The development of emotional intelligence becomes a powerful tool for navigating relationships with empathy and resilience.

Recognizing Behavioral Patterns
Behavioral patterns within toxic relationships often become entrenched and automatic. This subsection prompts individuals to recognize and dissect these

patterns with a keen self-awareness. Through self-observation and reflection, readers gain clarity on the behaviors that contribute to toxic dynamics, empowering them to interrupt and redirect these patterns towards healthier alternatives.

The Connection Between Self-Awareness and Healing
At the intersection of self-awareness and healing lies the potential for profound transformation. This section explores how self-awareness becomes a catalyst for healing, allowing individuals to break free from the shackles of toxic relationships. By fostering a compassionate understanding of oneself, readers cultivate the resilience needed to navigate the recovery journey with authenticity and grace.

Through the meticulous exploration of the power of self-awareness, individuals lay the foundation for breaking free from the confines of toxic relationships, fortifying themselves with the strength needed for the chapters of healing and renewal that follow.

Chapter 3: Detoxifying Your Mindset

Within the profound journey of breaking free from toxic relationships, the pivotal Chapter 3 serves as a compass for detoxifying the mindset – a transformative process that empowers men to reclaim control, foster resilience, and cultivate a positive and growth-oriented perspective. This chapter is a meticulous exploration into the intricate layers of mindset detoxification, offering tools and insights that guide individuals towards emotional strength and a renewed sense of self.

3.1 Challenging Negative Beliefs

Negative beliefs often take root in the fertile ground of toxic relationships, shaping perceptions and influencing self-worth. This section initiates a comprehensive examination into the process of challenging these negative beliefs. Through guided introspection and cognitive reframing exercises, individuals confront distorted thought patterns, gaining the tools to challenge and replace negative beliefs with affirming and empowering narratives.

Identifying and Examining Negative Beliefs
To challenge negative beliefs, individuals must first identify and examine the deep-seated narratives that have taken root within their minds. This subsection guides readers through the process of self-inquiry, prompting them to recognize and question the negative beliefs that may have been ingrained during the course of the toxic relationship. This critical step sets the stage for the subsequent process of transformation.

Cognitive Reframing Techniques
Cognitive reframing serves as a powerful tool for shifting perspectives and dismantling negative beliefs. This part introduces individuals to cognitive reframing techniques, providing practical strategies for reinterpreting challenging

situations and altering the associated beliefs. Through the intentional reshaping of thought patterns, readers pave the way for a more positive and constructive mindset.

Affirmations and Positive Reinforcement
Affirmations and positive reinforcement become anchors in the process of challenging negative beliefs. This subsection explores the transformative impact of incorporating positive affirmations into daily practices. Readers learn how to craft personalized affirmations that counteract negativity and reinforce a mindset aligned with self-empowerment and resilience.

3.2 Building Resilience and Emotional Strength

The toxic fallout from relationships often leaves individuals emotionally battered and depleted. This section of the chapter focuses on building resilience and emotional strength – essential components for navigating the path of recovery.

Understanding Resilience as a Skill
Resilience is not merely a trait; it is a skill that can be cultivated and strengthened. This subsection delves into the concept of resilience, exploring how individuals can develop the capacity to bounce back from adversity. Through resilience-building exercises and real-life examples, readers gain insights into the practical application of resilience as a skill within their own lives.

Embracing Emotional Strength
Emotional strength becomes a beacon in the process of detoxifying the mindset. This part guides individuals in embracing their emotional strength, acknowledging vulnerabilities, and fostering a compassionate relationship with their own emotions. Strategies for coping with emotional challenges and embracing vulnerability as a source of strength are explored in depth.

3.3 Cultivating a Positive and Growth-Oriented Mindset

The final leg of this transformative journey focuses on cultivating a positive and growth-oriented mindset. This section serves as the culmination of mindset detoxification, inviting individuals to embrace a perspective that fosters personal growth, resilience, and a hopeful outlook on the future.

The Power of Positivity
Positivity becomes a guiding force in the recovery journey. This subsection explores the impact of cultivating a positive mindset on overall well-being. Through gratitude practices, mindfulness, and intentional focus on positive aspects, individuals embark on a journey that reshapes their outlook and anchors them in a more optimistic frame of mind.

Embracing Growth Mindset Principles
A growth mindset becomes a cornerstone for embracing challenges as opportunities for learning and development. This part introduces the principles of a growth mindset, guiding individuals in adopting a perspective that views setbacks as stepping stones and failures as opportunities for growth. Through reflective exercises, readers internalize these principles, laying the foundation for a mindset that thrives on continuous learning and resilience.

Chapter 4: Cutting Ties - *Strategies for Ending Toxic Relationships*

In the profound odyssey of liberating oneself from the shackles of toxic relationships, Chapter 4 emerges as a pivotal guide, beckoning individuals to embark on the courageous journey of severing ties. This chapter represents a comprehensive exploration into the strategic process of disentangling from toxic relationships, presenting men with an arsenal of tools and profound insights essential for navigating this delicate phase. It is a transformative endeavor, ensuring resilience, safety, and an unyielding commitment to one's well-being.

4.1 Creating a Safe Exit Plan: Illuminating the Path to Freedom

The initiation of the journey towards freedom necessitates careful planning and a meticulous approach. This section serves as a beacon, guiding individuals in creating a safe exit plan that serves as a roadmap for their departure. It is a strategic endeavor designed to prioritize immediate safety and foster long-term well-being.

Assessing the Immediate Safety Concerns: A Critical First Step
At the forefront of creating a safe exit plan lies the imperative to assess immediate safety concerns. This subsection lays the groundwork for individuals to keenly identify potential risks and threats that may accompany the decision to sever ties. It's a critical first step, fostering a deep understanding of the urgency and gravity of the situation, allowing individuals to make decisions that safeguard their immediate well-being.

Securing Personal Documents and Resources: The Practical Aspects of Liberation
Leaving a toxic relationship involves practical considerations. This part of the

chapter delves into securing personal documents and resources, ensuring that individuals are equipped with the essentials for their journey to independence. It offers guidance on creating a checklist of necessary items, ensuring a smooth and practical transition as individuals prepare to break free from the constraints of toxic dynamics.

Identifying Safe Spaces and Support Networks: Fortifying the Emotional Foundations

Creating a safe exit plan extends beyond the physical logistics; it involves identifying safe spaces and establishing support networks. This subsection is a heartfelt guide, assisting individuals in pinpointing trusted friends, family members, or safe havens where they can find refuge during the exit process. It emphasizes the importance of emotional support, fortifying individuals with the resilience needed to navigate this challenging phase.

4.2 Establishing No-Contact Boundaries: Embracing the Power of Emotional Detox

Once the decision to sever ties is made, the establishment and maintenance of no-contact boundaries become paramount for emotional detoxification. This section explores the intricacies of creating firm and effective boundaries, shielding individuals from potential harm and facilitating the healing process.

Communicating Boundaries Clearly and Firmly: The Art of Assertiveness
Establishing no-contact boundaries commences with clear and firm communication. This subsection provides guidance on effectively articulating boundaries to the toxic partner. It is an exploration of assertiveness, emphasizing the need for clarity, conviction, and a steadfast commitment to the decision. Readers are equipped with the tools to navigate potential challenges, ensuring the boundaries are understood and respected.

Blocking Communication Channels: Technological Safeguards

Practical steps in enforcing no-contact boundaries involve blocking communication channels. This part explores the various methods individuals can employ to limit or block communication with the toxic partner, minimizing the potential for manipulation or coercion. Technological strategies, such as blocking phone numbers and social media accounts, are discussed to empower readers in maintaining their boundaries.

Coping with Emotional Challenges of No Contact: Nurturing Inner Resilience

Establishing no-contact boundaries can evoke a range of emotions, from guilt to sadness and even anxiety. This subsection delves into the emotional challenges associated with no contact, providing strategies for coping with these feelings. Readers gain insights into self-care practices, mindfulness techniques, and seeking support to navigate the emotional complexities of this phase, nurturing inner resilience.

4.3 Seeking Support from Friends, Family, and Professionals: Building a Fortress of Empathy

The aftermath of ending a toxic relationship is not a journey meant to be traversed alone. This section highlights the vital role of seeking support from friends, family, and professionals in fortifying individuals with the empathy and understanding needed for healing and renewal.

Building a Support Network: The Strength in Connection
Building a support network involves reaching out to trusted friends and family members who can provide emotional support and understanding. This subsection is a guide to identifying and connecting with individuals who can offer empathy, encouragement, and a non-judgmental

space during the challenging aftermath of ending a toxic relationship.

Professional Assistance and Counseling: Navigating the Complexities with Expert Guidance
Professional assistance becomes a valuable resource for those navigating the aftermath of a toxic relationship. This part introduces the benefits of seeking counseling or therapy to address the emotional fallout and provide a structured space for healing. Guidance on finding qualified professionals and resources for mental health support is explored, empowering individuals in their recovery journey.

Establishing Boundaries with Mutual Connections: Securing a Supportive Environment
To mitigate potential complications, individuals may need to establish boundaries with mutual connections, such as shared friends or acquaintances. This

subsection provides strategies for communicating boundaries to mutual connections, ensuring a supportive and respectful environment as individuals navigate the aftermath of the relationship.

It is a comprehensive guide, carefully crafted to navigate the delicate and strategic process of cutting ties with toxic relationships. Through the creation of a safe exit plan, the establishment of no-contact boundaries, and the strategic seeking of support, individuals lay the foundation for a transformative journey towards healing, resilience, and a renewed sense of autonomy. In this courageous chapter, the path to freedom is illuminated, and the seeds of renewal are sown.

Part II: Healing and Recovery

Chapter 5: Emotional Recovery - Nurturing the Seeds of Renewal

As individuals navigate the challenging terrain of healing and recovery following the aftermath of toxic relationships, Part II emerges as a sanctuary—a refuge where the process of rejuvenation unfolds. Within this sacred space, Chapter 5 takes center stage, serving as a guiding beacon for men embarking on the intricate journey of emotional recovery.

This pivotal chapter represents a profound exploration, seamlessly blending compassionate insights with empowering tools designed to navigate the complex emotional landscape that follows toxic relationships. Chapter 5 becomes a transformative experience, offering comprehensive guidance on processing grief and loss, understanding and managing anger, and reconstructing trust—both in oneself and in others.

Embarking on a Journey of Emotional Recovery

As men step into the realm of emotional recovery within the sanctuary of Chapter 5, they embark on a transformative journey that acknowledges the profound impact of toxic relationships on the emotional well-being. This chapter becomes a companion, a steadfast ally in navigating the intricate nuances of healing, providing a roadmap to traverse the varied emotional terrain with resilience and self-empowerment.

Processing Grief and Loss: Navigating the Depths of Heartache

The initial section of Chapter 5 delicately addresses the poignant process of processing grief and loss. It recognizes that toxic relationships leave behind a trail of emotional wreckage, prompting individuals to confront and navigate the depths of heartache. Through thoughtful insights and practical tools, this exploration encourages a comprehensive understanding of grief's layers, fostering a healing environment where individuals can confront and release the emotional burden carried from the toxic past.

Understanding and Managing Anger: Channeling Emotion into Empowerment
The exploration then seamlessly transitions into the intricate landscape of anger—an emotion often intensified in the aftermath of toxic relationships. Chapter 5 serves as a guide for understanding and managing anger, providing individuals with the necessary tools to transform this potent emotion into a catalyst for empowerment. By delving into the roots of anger, the chapter enables a constructive expression of this emotion, promoting a healthier emotional state.

*Rebuilding Trust in Oneself and Others:
The Architecture of Renewal*

The culminating section of Chapter 5 addresses the pivotal theme of rebuilding trust—an essential pillar in the architecture of renewal. Recognizing the profound impact of shattered trust in toxic relationships, this exploration becomes a compass, guiding individuals in reconstructing trust in oneself and others. By laying the groundwork for self-trust and offering strategies to navigate the delicate process of trusting others, the chapter empowers individuals to rebuild a foundation that supports renewed self-belief and healthier interpersonal connections.

An Invitation to Transformation and Empowerment

Chapter 5 extends an invitation—a beckoning call to transformation and empowerment. It is not merely a chapter but a sanctuary within the larger narrative of healing. Here, individuals find solace, understanding, and actionable tools to navigate the intricate dance of emotions that follow toxic relationships. This chapter stands as a testament to resilience, an affirmation that, even in the face of emotional turmoil, there exists a path to rejuvenation. As men engage with the content within this sanctuary of emotional recovery, they discover the transformative power that lies within their grasp—an empowerment that leads to renewal, healing, and the reclamation of emotional well-being.

5.1 Processing Grief and Loss: Navigating the Landscape of Heartache

The aftermath of a toxic relationship often leaves behind a landscape of heartache and grief. This section of Chapter 5 is a compassionate guide, leading individuals through the delicate process of processing grief and loss. It acknowledges the depth of emotional pain and provides tools to navigate the intricate terrain of healing.

Recognizing the Layers of Grief
Grief is a multi-faceted emotion, and recognizing its layers is the first step towards healing. This subsection explores the various dimensions of grief that may accompany the end of a toxic relationship. From the loss of trust to shattered dreams, readers gain insights into the diverse facets of grief, creating a roadmap for understanding and addressing these complex emotions.

Embracing the Grieving Process
Embracing the grieving process becomes an essential component of emotional recovery. This part guides individuals through the stages of grief, offering insights into the emotional landscape that accompanies each phase. By embracing grief as a natural and necessary part of healing, readers lay the

foundation for a transformative journey towards renewal.

Rituals of Closure and Release

Closure is a profound need in the aftermath of a toxic relationship, and rituals can be powerful tools for achieving it. This subsection explores the concept of closure rituals, offering suggestions for meaningful practices that allow individuals to symbolically release the pain and baggage associated with the toxic dynamics. From writing letters to symbolic gestures, readers discover personalized ways to foster closure and release.

5.2 Understanding and Managing Anger: Harnessing the Power of Emotion

Anger is a potent and often complex emotion that can emerge as individuals grapple with the aftermath of toxic relationships. This section of Chapter 5 is a guide to understanding and managing anger, providing strategies to harness this powerful emotion constructively.

Unpacking the Roots of Anger
Anger, often a surface emotion, conceals deeper roots that need exploration. This subsection encourages individuals to unpack the roots of their anger, delving into the underlying emotions and triggers that fuel this intense response. By understanding the source of anger, readers gain insights into the complexities of their emotional landscape.

Constructive Expression of Anger
Rather than suppressing or succumbing to destructive expressions, this part explores the importance of constructive outlets for anger. From journaling to physical activities, readers discover ways to channel their anger in healthy and productive ways. This section is a roadmap to transforming anger into a catalyst for personal growth and empowerment.

Seeking Professional Guidance for Anger Management

For those grappling with intense anger, seeking professional guidance becomes an invaluable resource. This subsection introduces the benefits of anger management counseling or therapy, providing individuals with the tools and support needed to navigate and transform this powerful emotion. It emphasizes the importance of seeking help as a proactive step towards emotional recovery.

5.3 Rebuilding Trust in Yourself and Others: The Architecture of Renewal

Trust, once shattered, becomes a cornerstone in the process of rebuilding oneself. Chapter 5's exploration culminates in guiding individuals through the intricate journey of rebuilding trust in oneself and others. This section is a profound exploration, offering strategies to mend the fractures of trust and construct a resilient foundation for renewed self-belief.

Self-Trust as a Fundamental Pillar
Rebuilding trust begins with self-trust, and this subsection delves into the intricate process of restoring faith in oneself. It guides individuals through self-reflective practices and exercises, fostering a compassionate relationship with the self. By acknowledging personal strengths and achievements, readers lay the groundwork for rebuilding the fundamental pillar of self-trust.

Navigating the Path to Trusting Others
Trusting others after the turmoil of a toxic relationship requires a cautious yet open-hearted approach. This part explores strategies for navigating the path to trusting others, offering insights into setting healthy boundaries, communication, and discernment. Readers gain tools to distinguish between red flags and genuine

connections, fostering a gradual yet intentional rebuilding of trust in interpersonal relationships.

Professional Support in Trust Restoration
For those navigating the complex terrain of trust restoration, seeking professional support becomes an invaluable resource. This subsection introduces the benefits of therapy or counseling in rebuilding trust, providing individuals with a structured space to explore past traumas, develop coping strategies, and cultivate the skills needed for trusting oneself and others. It underscores the importance of professional guidance as a foundational element in the architecture of renewal.

As men engage with the content of this Chapter, they embark on a transformative journey of emotional recovery. It is a sanctuary where the seeds of renewal are nurtured, and the intricacies of grief, anger, and trust are explored with compassion and wisdom. Through processing grief and loss, understanding and managing anger, and rebuilding trust in oneself and others, individuals lay the foundation for a resilient and empowered emotional recovery. In this pivotal chapter, the landscape of healing unfolds, and the journey towards renewal takes a profound and compassionate form.

Chapter 6: Rebuilding Self-Esteem and Confidence - A Journey to Self-Rediscovery

In the transformative odyssey of recovering from toxic relationships, Chapter 6 emerges as a guiding light—a beacon illuminating the path to rebuilding self-esteem and confidence. This chapter is a profound exploration into the intricate process of self-rediscovery, offering a comprehensive guide to men seeking to reclaim their sense of self-worth and confidence. With a focus on embracing self-compassion, setting realistic goals for personal growth, and rediscovering strengths and talents, Chapter 6 becomes a transformative sanctuary within the larger narrative of healing and renewal.

6.1 Embracing Self-Compassion: Nurturing the Seed of Self-Love

At the heart of rebuilding self-esteem and confidence lies the crucial element of self-compassion. This section of Chapter 6 is a compassionate journey into the art of embracing oneself with kindness and understanding. Recognizing that individuals emerging from toxic relationships often carry wounds of self-criticism, this exploration delves into practices and perspectives that nurture the seed of self-love.

Understanding the Essence of Self-Compassion
This subsection lays the foundation for embracing self-compassion by delving into its essence. Readers are guided to understand the components of self-compassion, which include self-kindness, common humanity, and mindfulness. Through relatable examples and practical exercises, individuals learn to cultivate a gentler and more supportive inner dialogue.

Practices for Cultivating Self-Compassion
Turning theory into practice, this part offers actionable strategies for cultivating self-compassion. From mindfulness exercises to self-affirmations, individuals are equipped with tools to shift from self-criticism to self-acceptance. The exploration encourages a nurturing environment where men learn to extend the same understanding and empathy to themselves that they may readily offer to others.

6.2 Setting Realistic Goals for Personal Growth: Paving the Path to Empowerment

As individuals begin to embrace self-compassion, the journey into rebuilding self-esteem continues with a focus on setting realistic goals for personal growth. This section becomes a roadmap—a guide for men to pave the path towards empowerment by establishing achievable and meaningful objectives for their individual journey.

Identifying Personal Values and Aspirations
Setting realistic goals starts with a deep understanding of personal values and aspirations. This subsection encourages individuals to reflect on their core values, passions, and aspirations, laying the groundwork for goals that align with their authentic selves. By aligning goals with personal values, individuals establish a foundation for sustained motivation and fulfillment.

Creating Incremental Steps Towards Growth
Realistic goals are often achieved through incremental steps. This part introduces the concept of breaking down larger goals into manageable tasks, fostering a sense of accomplishment with each step forward. Through practical strategies and examples, individuals learn to create a roadmap for

personal growth that celebrates progress and builds confidence.

Adapting Goals to Changing Circumstances
The journey of personal growth is dynamic, and goals may need adjustments along the way. This subsection guides individuals in adapting their goals to changing circumstances with flexibility and resilience. It emphasizes the importance of self-reflection and the ability to recalibrate objectives in alignment with evolving personal needs and aspirations.

6.3 Rediscovering Your Strengths and Talents: Unveiling the Authentic Self

The final phase of Chapter 6 invites individuals to embark on a journey of rediscovering their strengths and talents—a pivotal aspect of rebuilding self-esteem. This exploration becomes a mirror reflecting the authentic self, helping men uncover and celebrate the unique qualities that contribute to their sense of worth and confidence.

Reflecting on Personal Achievements and Resilience
The process of rediscovery begins with reflection. This subsection encourages individuals to reflect on their personal achievements and moments of resilience. By acknowledging past triumphs, individuals gain a deeper appreciation for their strengths and resilience, laying the groundwork for rebuilding self-esteem.

Exploring Untapped Talents and Passions
Rediscovering strengths extends to exploring untapped talents and passions. This part invites individuals to step outside their comfort zones, try new activities, and reconnect with hobbies or interests that may have been overshadowed in toxic relationships. Through exploration, men uncover hidden facets of themselves, fostering a renewed sense of self-worth.

Integrating Strengths and Talents into Daily Life

The final subsection offers practical guidance on integrating rediscovered strengths and talents into daily life. Individuals are empowered to weave these authentic elements into their routines, relationships, and personal pursuits. This integration becomes a testament to the journey of self-rediscovery, transforming daily experiences into opportunities for empowerment and growth.

As we digest the transformative content of Chapter 6, we embark on a journey of self-rediscovery—a journey that transcends the scars of toxic relationships and leads to the emergence of a more resilient, empowered, and confident self. Through embracing self-compassion, setting realistic goals for personal growth, and rediscovering strengths and talents, this chapter becomes a sanctuary for the reclamation of self-esteem and confidence. It is a pivotal step in the larger narrative of healing—a testament to the transformative power of self-love, personal growth, and the authentic unveiling of one's true potential.

Chapter 7: Forgiveness - The Key to Liberation

In the profound journey of healing and recovery, Chapter 7 emerges as a poignant exploration into the transformative power of forgiveness—a key to liberation from the emotional chains of toxic relationships. This chapter serves as a guide, delving into the intricate facets of forgiveness, encompassing the transformative power it holds, the complexities of forgiving oneself and others, and the liberating act of letting go of resentment and embracing the path forward.

7.1 The Transformative Power of Forgiveness: Unshackling Emotional Chains

The exploration begins with an in-depth understanding of the transformative power inherent in forgiveness. Chapter 7 unveils forgiveness as a profound act of liberation, capable of unshackling the emotional chains that bind individuals to the pain of past toxic relationships. It delves into the psychology of forgiveness, highlighting its ability to release resentment and pave the way for inner peace and emotional freedom.

Understanding the Psychology of Forgiveness
This subsection illuminates the psychological dimensions of forgiveness, exploring the cognitive and emotional shifts that occur when individuals embark on the journey of forgiving. It introduces concepts such as empathy, compassion, and the rewiring of negative thought patterns, offering readers a comprehensive understanding of the transformative processes at play.

The Physical and Emotional Benefits of Forgiveness
Forgiveness transcends the emotional realm, extending its impact to physical and mental well-being. This part delves into the tangible benefits of forgiveness, from stress reduction and improved immune function to

enhanced mental health. It becomes a compelling exploration, underscoring the holistic nature of forgiveness and its potential to unlock a path to overall well-being.

Cultivating a Forgiving Mindset
The journey into forgiveness involves cultivating a forgiving mindset—a way of thinking that fosters understanding and compassion. This subsection offers practical strategies and exercises to help individuals shift their mindset toward forgiveness. It becomes a guide to reshaping perspectives, nurturing empathy, and creating a mental space conducive to the transformative power of forgiveness.

7.2 Forgiving Yourself and Others: The Compassionate Act of Release

Forgiveness extends beyond external relationships, encompassing the intricate dance of forgiving oneself and others. This section of Chapter 7 becomes a compassionate guide, exploring the complexities and nuances involved in the liberating act of forgiveness.

The Liberation of Forgiving Oneself
The journey of self-forgiveness is often the first step towards liberation. This subsection navigates the intricacies of forgiving oneself, addressing self-blame, guilt, and shame. Through self-compassion exercises and reflective practices, individuals embark on a transformative journey of releasing the burdens of the past and fostering a renewed sense of self-acceptance.

Extending Compassion to Others
Forgiving others becomes a profound act of extending compassion beyond oneself. This part explores the challenges and rewards of forgiving those who have caused pain. It provides practical tools for navigating the complexities of interpersonal forgiveness, emphasizing the role of empathy,

understanding, and intentional release in fostering emotional healing.

Rebuilding Relationships Through Forgiveness

Forgiveness holds the potential to rebuild relationships tainted by toxicity. This subsection delves into the dynamics of rebuilding connections through forgiveness, offering insights into effective communication, setting boundaries, and cultivating a shared commitment to healing. It becomes a guide for those seeking to transform fractured relationships into spaces of understanding, growth, and mutual respect.

7.3 Letting Go of Resentment and Moving Forward: Embracing the Path Ahead

The final segment of Chapter 7 invites individuals to let go of resentment—an act that marks the culmination of the forgiveness journey. This section becomes a roadmap to moving forward, embracing the path ahead with newfound emotional freedom and a sense of liberation.

Releasing Resentment: The Liberation Ritual

The act of letting go is a symbolic and transformative ritual. This subsection offers practical exercises and rituals for releasing resentment, allowing individuals to consciously and intentionally unburden themselves from the weight of past grievances. It becomes a liberating ceremony, marking a shift from pain to freedom.

Embracing the Path Forward: Cultivating Resilience

Moving forward after forgiveness requires the cultivation of resilience. This part explores strategies for building emotional resilience, emphasizing self-care, mindfulness, and ongoing personal growth. It becomes a guide to navigating the uncertainties of the future with strength, grace, and an empowered sense of self.

The Ongoing Journey of Forgiveness: Nurturing Emotional Freedom
The forgiveness journey is ongoing, and this subsection acknowledges the continuous nature of forgiveness. It becomes an invitation to nurture emotional freedom through ongoing practices, reflection, and a commitment to the principles of forgiveness. Individuals are encouraged to embrace forgiveness as a lifelong journey—a path that leads to sustained liberation and well-being.

Engaging with the contents of this Chapter , we embark on a profound exploration of forgiveness—a key that unlocks the door to emotional liberation. This chapter becomes a sanctuary for those seeking to release the shackles of resentment, both towards themselves and others, and embrace a future defined by compassion, understanding, and the transformative power of forgiveness. It is a pivotal step in the larger narrative of healing—a testament to the strength found in letting go and the liberation that forgiveness brings to the intricate tapestry of one's emotional landscape.

Part III: Thriving After Toxicity

Chapter 8: Healthy Relationship Dynamics - Cultivating Flourishing Connections

As individuals transition from the shadows of toxic relationships into the realm of thriving, Part III unfolds as a compass guiding them towards a life characterized by healthy relationship dynamics. Chapter 8 stands as a beacon within this transformative journey, offering a comprehensive exploration of recognizing, cultivating, and sustaining flourishing connections.

From understanding and fostering healthy relationship traits to setting and communicating boundaries, and nurturing mutual respect and empathy, this chapter becomes a roadmap to not just recovery but the cultivation of thriving relationships.

8.1 Recognizing and Cultivating Healthy Relationship Traits: The Foundation of Flourishing Connections

The initial section of Chapter 8 serves as a foundational exploration, delving into the intricacies of recognizing and cultivating healthy relationship traits. It becomes a guide to identifying the building blocks that contribute to the vitality of connections, empowering individuals to foster and sustain relationships that contribute positively to their well-being.

Identifying Positive Communication Patterns

Communication lies at the heart of healthy relationships. This subsection explores positive communication patterns, emphasizing active listening, constructive dialogue, and open expression of thoughts and emotions. It becomes a guide to fostering an environment where individuals feel heard, understood, and valued—a crucial aspect of cultivating flourishing connections.

Embracing Emotional Intelligence
Emotional intelligence becomes a cornerstone in healthy relationships. This part delves into the components of emotional intelligence, encouraging individuals to recognize and regulate their emotions while fostering empathy towards others. Through self-awareness and understanding, individuals pave the way for connections that thrive on mutual understanding and emotional resonance.

Fostering Trust and Transparency
Trust forms the bedrock of healthy relationships. This subsection explores the dynamics of trust and transparency, guiding individuals to foster an environment where trust can flourish. It becomes a roadmap to navigating the delicate balance between openness and privacy, creating connections

built on a foundation of honesty and reliability.

8.2 Setting and Communicating Boundaries: Nurturing Individual Autonomy

The journey towards healthy relationship dynamics continues with a focus on setting and communicating boundaries. This section becomes a guide to establishing a framework that nurtures individual autonomy while fostering connection—a delicate balance that ensures relationships thrive on mutual respect and understanding.

Understanding the Importance of Boundaries
This subsection delves into the significance of boundaries in relationships, emphasizing their role in preserving individual autonomy and emotional well-being. It becomes a guide for individuals to understand and

articulate their personal boundaries, fostering a sense of agency and empowerment within the dynamics of connections.

Communicating Boundaries Effectively
Setting boundaries is only part of the equation; effective communication is equally crucial. This part offers practical strategies for communicating boundaries in a clear, respectful, and assertive manner. Through open dialogue, individuals establish a shared understanding of each other's needs, cultivating an environment where boundaries are acknowledged and respected.

Navigating Challenges and Adjusting Boundaries
The exploration extends to navigating challenges that may arise in maintaining boundaries. This subsection provides insights into handling conflicts, adjusting boundaries when necessary, and fostering a

culture of adaptability within relationships. It becomes a guide for individuals to navigate the evolving dynamics of connections with resilience and open communication.

8.3 Nurturing Mutual Respect and Empathy: The Heartbeat of Flourishing Connections

The final segment of Chapter 8 invites individuals to nurture mutual respect and empathy—an essential heartbeat that sustains flourishing connections. This section becomes a guide to fostering an environment where understanding, compassion, and a genuine regard for each other's well-being become the pillars upon which relationships flourish.

Cultivating Active Empathy
Empathy becomes a powerful tool in healthy relationships. This subsection explores the nuances of active empathy, guiding individuals to step into each other's shoes,

understand perspectives, and respond with compassion. Through empathy, connections deepen, and a culture of mutual understanding blossoms.

Prioritizing Mutual Well-Being
The reciprocal nature of healthy relationships places a premium on mutual well-being. This part encourages individuals to prioritize the health and happiness of both themselves and their partners. It becomes a guide for fostering an environment where each person's growth, fulfillment, and happiness are integral to the fabric of the relationship.

Celebrating Differences and Individual Growth
Flourishing connections embrace the uniqueness of individuals within the relationship. This subsection explores the art of celebrating differences and supporting each other's individual growth. It becomes a guide to creating a dynamic where diversity

is valued, and the journey of personal development is celebrated as a shared endeavor within the relationship.

Chapter 9: Building a Supportive Network - Nurturing Connections for Recovery

As individuals embark on the journey of recovery and growth, Chapter 9 unfolds as a vital exploration into building a supportive network—a web of connections designed to fortify and uplift during the process of healing.

This chapter becomes a comprehensive guide, addressing the nuances of establishing meaningful connections, the benefits of seeking professional counseling and therapy, and the transformative power of joining support groups specifically tailored for men in recovery. It stands as a beacon within the larger narrative, offering a roadmap to construct a robust and nurturing support system that becomes a cornerstone in the recovery journey.

9.1 Establishing Meaningful Connections: The Foundation of Support

The foundational section of Chapter 9 delves into the art of establishing meaningful connections. It becomes a guide for individuals seeking to construct a support network that goes beyond mere association, fostering relationships that are genuine, understanding, and integral to the journey of recovery.

Identifying and Nurturing Positive Relationships

This subsection explores the process of identifying positive relationships and nurturing them for mutual growth. It offers insights into recognizing the characteristics of supportive individuals, fostering connections based on empathy, trust, and shared values. Through intentional cultivation, individuals lay the groundwork for a support system that becomes a pillar of strength in times of need.

Communicating Needs and Establishing Boundaries

Effective communication forms the linchpin of meaningful connections. This part delves into the importance of communicating needs and establishing boundaries within relationships. It becomes a guide for individuals to express their requirements, set expectations, and foster an environment where support flows seamlessly while respecting individual boundaries.

The Reciprocity of Support: Giving and Receiving

Meaningful connections thrive on reciprocity—the give-and-take of support. This subsection explores the dynamics of supporting others within the network while also being open to receiving support when needed. It becomes a guide to cultivating a culture of mutual assistance and understanding within the supportive network, fostering an environment of shared resilience.

9.2 Seeking Professional Counseling and Therapy: The Guiding Hand of Expert Support

The journey of recovery often benefits immensely from the professional guidance offered by counseling and therapy. This section becomes a comprehensive exploration into the transformative power of seeking professional support, providing individuals with the tools and insights necessary to navigate the complexities of their emotions and experiences.

Recognizing the Role of Professional Support in Recovery

This subsection elucidates the crucial role that professional counseling and therapy play in the recovery process. It explores the benefits of seeking expert guidance, from gaining a deeper understanding of personal challenges to receiving tailored strategies for coping and growth. It becomes a guide for individuals to recognize the value of professional support as a guiding hand through the intricacies of their unique recovery journey.

Finding the Right Counselor or Therapist
The process of seeking professional support begins with finding the right counselor or therapist. This part offers practical advice on selecting professionals whose expertise aligns with individual needs and goals. It becomes a guide for navigating the process of establishing a therapeutic relationship, ensuring a harmonious and effective collaboration towards recovery.

Incorporating Therapy into the Recovery Plan
Therapy becomes a dynamic component within the larger recovery plan. This subsection explores the integration of therapeutic interventions into the overall recovery strategy, emphasizing the synergistic relationship between self-reflection, professional guidance, and personal growth. It becomes a guide to

maximizing the benefits of therapy as a transformative tool in the journey towards holistic recovery.

9.3 Joining Support Groups for Men in Recovery: Community and Connection

The final segment of Chapter 9 explores the transformative power of joining support groups specifically tailored for men in recovery. It becomes a guide to leveraging the strength of communal understanding, shared experiences, and a collective commitment to growth within a supportive group dynamic.

The Importance of Gender-Specific Support
This subsection delves into the significance of gender-specific support groups, particularly tailored for men. It explores the unique challenges men may face in the recovery process, providing a safe and understanding space for open discussions. It becomes a guide for individuals to connect

with others who share similar experiences, fostering a sense of camaraderie and shared strength.

The Dynamics of Group Support
Joining a support group introduces individuals to the dynamics of collective support. This part explores the benefits of group interactions, from shared insights and encouragement to the validation of personal experiences. It becomes a guide to navigating the group dynamic, contributing and receiving support in a collaborative environment that promotes healing and growth.

Sustaining Long-Term Connections
The journey of recovery extends beyond immediate challenges, and support groups become a long-term network. This subsection provides insights into sustaining connections forged within the group, fostering enduring relationships that contribute to ongoing resilience and growth.

It becomes a guide to the cultivation of a supportive community that remains steadfast in the face of evolving personal journeys.

Chapter 10: Creating a Life of Fulfillment - The Culmination of Recovery

As individuals progress through the transformative journey of recovery, Chapter 10 unfolds as a poignant exploration into the creation of a life filled with fulfillment. This chapter becomes a comprehensive guide, addressing the pursuit of passion and purpose, the delicate balance between work, relationships, and personal well-being, and the celebration of the remarkable journey of recovery. It stands as a culmination within the larger narrative, offering a roadmap to not only reclaiming one's life but sculpting it into a tapestry of joy, purpose, and genuine fulfillment.

10.1 Pursuing Passion and Purpose: The Heartbeat of a Fulfilling Life

The initial section of Chapter 10 delves into the profound exploration of pursuing passion and purpose—a fundamental aspect of creating a life filled with fulfillment. It becomes a guide for individuals to rediscover their passions, align with their purpose, and infuse every aspect of their lives with a sense of meaning and direction.

Uncovering Personal Passions
This subsection guides individuals on a journey of self-discovery, encouraging them to uncover and embrace their personal passions. It becomes a roadmap to reconnecting with activities, interests, and pursuits that bring genuine joy and fulfillment. Through introspection and exploration, individuals reignite the flames of passion that may have dimmed during the challenges of toxic relationships.

Aligning with Purpose
Passion gains its fullest expression when aligned with purpose. This part explores the intersection of passion and purpose, guiding individuals to identify the values, causes, or

missions that resonate deeply with their authentic selves. It becomes a guide to infusing purpose into daily life, creating a foundation for a fulfilling and meaningful existence.

Integrating Passion and Purpose into Daily Life
The pursuit of passion and purpose extends beyond discovery; it involves integration into daily life. This subsection provides practical strategies for seamlessly weaving passion and purpose into various aspects of life, from career choices to personal relationships. It becomes a guide for individuals to cultivate a life where each day is infused with the energy and fulfillment derived from living authentically.

10.2 Balancing Work, Relationships, and Personal Well-being: The Harmony of a Fulfilling Life

The journey towards a fulfilling life encompasses the delicate art of balance—balancing work, relationships, and personal well-being. This section becomes a comprehensive exploration into the dynamics of creating harmony within these essential facets, ensuring that each contributes positively to the overall tapestry of a satisfying and well-rounded life.

Navigating Work-Life Balance
Work, while a crucial aspect of life, requires a harmonious balance to prevent burnout and foster overall well-being. This subsection explores strategies for navigating work-life balance, from setting boundaries and managing priorities to fostering a workplace environment that supports personal fulfillment. It becomes a guide to crafting a career that aligns with individual

values and contributes positively to a fulfilling life.

Cultivating Healthy Relationships
Healthy relationships become a cornerstone of a fulfilling life. This part delves into the dynamics of cultivating and sustaining relationships that contribute positively to personal growth and well-being. It becomes a guide for navigating the intricacies of communication, emotional intimacy, and mutual support within relationships. Through intentional efforts, individuals foster connections that enhance rather than detract from the overall quality of life.

Prioritizing Personal Well-being
The pursuit of a fulfilling life necessitates prioritizing personal well-being. This subsection explores the importance of self-care, mindfulness, and intentional practices that nurture physical, mental, and emotional health. It becomes a guide to creating a well-rounded approach to

well-being, ensuring that individuals have the resilience and vitality to fully engage in the various dimensions of their lives.

10.3 Celebrating Your Journey of Recovery: Embracing Triumph and Growth

The final segment of Chapter 10 invites individuals to celebrate their remarkable journey of recovery. It becomes a guide to acknowledging triumphs, embracing growth, and cultivating a mindset of gratitude for the resilience displayed throughout the challenging yet transformative process of recovery.

Recognizing Personal Triumphs
This subsection prompts individuals to reflect on and recognize the personal triumphs achieved throughout their recovery journey. It becomes a guide to acknowledging resilience, courage, and the milestones that mark significant progress. Through this recognition, individuals

cultivate a sense of empowerment and self-appreciation.

Embracing Ongoing Growth
Recovery is a dynamic and ongoing process that involves continuous growth. This part explores the concept of embracing ongoing personal and emotional development, encouraging individuals to view growth as a lifelong journey. It becomes a guide to fostering a growth mindset, where challenges are viewed as opportunities for learning and self-improvement.

Cultivating a Mindset of Gratitude
Gratitude becomes a transformative lens through which to view one's journey. This subsection explores the cultivation of a mindset of gratitude, guiding individuals to appreciate the lessons learned, the strength gained, and the support received throughout the recovery process. It becomes a guide to fostering a positive outlook that enhances

the overall sense of fulfillment and well-being.

Conclusion: A Tapestry of Triumph and Renewal

In the concluding chapter, we find ourselves at the culmination of a transformative journey—a journey that has traversed the intricate terrain of toxic relationship recovery for men. This conclusion serves as a reflective vantage point, offering a panoramic view of the path traveled and the profound transformations experienced. It becomes a tapestry woven with the threads of triumph, resilience, renewal, and the unwavering commitment to reclaiming not only one's life but crafting a narrative of enduring fulfillment.

As we take a retrospective gaze, it is essential to acknowledge the depth of the challenges faced within toxic relationships. The complexities inherent in these dynamics often weave a web of emotional, mental, and sometimes physical struggles that can leave lasting imprints on an individual's well-being. The journey embarked upon in the preceding chapters has been an exploration into the heart of this complexity—a quest for understanding, healing, and renewal specifically tailored for the unique needs of men navigating the aftermath of toxic relationships.

From the initial chapters unraveling the intricate layers of toxic relationship dynamics to the profound insights into the impact on men's mental and emotional well-being, the journey has been one of illumination. It has provided a space for introspection, challenging societal expectations, and embracing the vulnerability necessary for authentic healing. The recognition that toxic relationships are not a testament to personal failure but a reflection of the intricacies within human connections has been a transformative paradigm shift—one that sets the stage for a renewed sense of self.

The chapters dedicated to breaking free and the power of self-reflection have been pivotal in empowering individuals to reassess their relationship dynamics, establish personal boundaries, and harness the transformative power of self-awareness. It is a testament to the strength found in self-discovery—a strength that forms the bedrock of recovery.

The exploration into the intricacies of emotional recovery, rebuilding self-esteem, and the transformative power of forgiveness has been a profound journey into the heart of emotional healing. It is a recognition that true recovery extends beyond the cessation of toxic dynamics—it involves the restoration of emotional well-being, the rebuilding of self-esteem, and the liberation found in forgiveness, both for oneself and others.

The chapters navigating the creation of a supportive network and fostering healthy relationships are not just guides but affirmations that connection is a fundamental element in the human experience. By establishing meaningful connections, seeking professional support when necessary, and engaging in supportive communities, individuals forge a network that becomes a wellspring of strength, understanding, and shared growth.

The exploration into creating a life of fulfillment is the crescendo of this transformative symphony. It is an invitation to pursue passion and purpose, balance work, relationships, and personal well-being, and celebrate the journey of recovery. This chapter serves as a testament to the resilience displayed, the growth achieved, and the potential for a life marked not only by the absence of toxicity but by the presence of genuine joy, purpose, and fulfillment.

As we conclude this transformative odyssey, it is imperative to recognize that the journey of recovery is not a linear path. It is a dynamic process marked by ebbs and flows, setbacks and triumphs, moments of vulnerability and profound strength. This conclusion is not an endpoint but a threshold—a threshold to a new beginning where individuals emerge not only as survivors but as architects of their own destinies.

In the symphony of recovery, every chapter, every exploration, and every revelation has played a crucial note—a note that contributes to the harmonious melody of renewal. This conclusion, therefore, is an affirmation that the journey towards healing is not merely a pursuit of recovery but a creation of a life imbued with resilience, authenticity, and enduring fulfillment.

May this conclusion be a compass guiding individuals beyond the pages of this narrative—a compass that points towards a future marked by the triumphant echoes of recovery and the vibrant hues of a life reconstructed with intention, purpose, and an unwavering commitment to thriving after toxicity.